The Best Guide To:

Intermittent Fasting Diet

Get in Shape and Lose Fat in 7 Days with this Incredible Weight Loss Intermittent Fasting Diet Plan!

I0428318

Chris Smith

STOP!!! Before you read any further....Would you like to know the Secrets of Body Transformation?

If your answer is yes, then you are not alone. Thousands of people are looking for the secret to rapidly burn body fat, keep the weight off, become healthier, and truly transform their body and life for good.

If you have been searching for these answers without much luck, you are in the right place!

Not only will you gain incredible insight in this book, but because I want to make sure to give you as much value as possible, right now for a limited time you can get full **100% FREE access to a VIP bonus EBook** entitled **THE 7 KEYS TO BODY TRANSFORMATION!**

Just Go Here For Free Instant Access:

www.liveFitVIP.com

Legal Notice

Disclaimer Notice

Table Of Contents

Introduction

I want to thank you and congratulate you for purchasing the book, "Intermittent Fasting Diet: The Best Guide to Intermittent Fasting - Get in Shape and Lose Fat in 7 Days with this Incredible Weight Loss Intermittent Fasting Diet Plan!".

This book contains proven steps and strategies on how Intermittent Fasting can not only help you lose fat rapidly, but keep it off for life!

Have you been working out consistently? Eating the recommended 4-6 meals each day? And still, you are unable to reveal your six pack and glutes to the world?

You are not alone. For years supplement companies, fitness magazines, bodybuilders, fitness trainers, health gurus, and many others have been all telling the same advice to lose fat and gain muscle. Their solution for your fitness goals - Eat 4-6 miniature chipmunk sized meals, do lots of weight training, and even more cardio. So, the time is now to ask yourself one simple question, "How's that working out for ya?".

If you don't feel too good about your fitness results, and really want to see that six pack, lean muscular physique, then you are reading the right book. The time is now to try the most revolutionary new diet, which I would rather refer to as a lifestyle - Intermittent Fasting!

Thanks again for purchasing this book, I hope you enjoy it!

Chapter 1 - Intermittent Fasting And Its Benefits

Intermittent fasting is markedly different from any other diet plan that you may have tried in the past. Most weight loss plans espoused by fitness gurus will tell you to control the amount you eat while keeping a close watch on the kinds of food that you do consume, usually in combination with a rigorous exercise routine. You know this: you've done the cardio, lifted the weights, run the miles, and eaten 6 small meals a day, all the while assiduously avoiding unhealthy fats and unnecessary carbohydrates.

But you are probably reading this book because this system just doesn't work for you – in fact, it has probably left you tired, crabby, and frustrated, with nothing to show for your hard work but a few insignificant inches shed from your waistline and some mad food cravings that are proving harder and harder to ignore.

This is not to say that typical diet programs don't work. After all, there's a reason why they have their staunch advocates. But the fact remains that for most people, it is much more effective – and much easier – to control when they eat, instead of what they eat and the portions thereof.

That's what intermittent fasting, also known as IF, is all about. To put it in the very simplest terms, when you adopt this lifestyle, you will only eat during a certain period of time daily, and go entirely without food, which is the fasting bitfor the rest of the day. That's all there is to it. And, once you consider the amount of time that there actually is between meals, you'll see that it isn't hard at all.

There is no denying that exercise and healthy eating are important (you can't hope to get that six-pack if you live on fast food burgers and stay on the couch all day, but more on that later), but intermittent fasting can work wonders on its own. Before we go on to the nitty-gritty of this fitness lifestyle, let's take a look at the unique benefits that it has to offer.

Better Weight Control and Faster Fat Loss

Since shedding pounds and losing inches are the most conspicuous signs of success of any diet program – not to mention your most likely objective when you start dieting –we'll start here. Intermittent fasting is exceptionally effective at helping you lose fat since it eases your body into a situation where it starts burning fat stores for energy. And since this will happen every single day that you go through a period of fasting, you will lose fat faster and have better control over your body weight than if you stick to counting calories.

Elimination of Pesky Food Cravings

One of the major trials for any dieter is the craving for snacks and sweets, and, admittedly, those will still be there when you start intermittent fasting. Once you get into the habit, however, you'll find that your pesky food cravings aren't troubling you as much, and soon you just won't feel them anymore. Scientists theorize that this is due to fasting bringing the level of your body's ghrelin, otherwise known as the "hunger hormone", down to normal, so you don't continually feel the urge to snack.

Reduced Oxidation with Boosted Autophagy

Oxidative stress caused by free radicals in your system can really take its toll on your body's cells. The damage done by free radicals to DNA, RNA, proteins, and lipids is known to advance the effects of aging and disease. Going on an intermittent fasting diet will help combat this by boosting autophagy, or the process by which cellular waste is recycled by your body. This helps your cells get rid of the trash, so to speak, so that they can continue to function optimally, allowing you to better withstand stress, disease, and aging.

A Healthier Nervous System and Mental Clarity

Though it is commonly believed that fasting will leave you weak and unable to think, nothing could be further from the truth. Intermittent fasting has actually been shown to enhance memory and learning, as well as helping to improve your disposition in life. This is because periodic fasting boosts the production of brain-derived neurotrophic factor (BDNF), a hormone that prevents the degradation of the neurons in your brain while stimulating the growth of new neurons. A boost in the neurotransmitter serotonin also happens, which leads to better moods and improved learning ability.

Enjoyable Longevity

While any sort of health and fitness regime has the long-term aim of prolonging your life, one of the main attractions of intermittent fasting for many people is that it promotes enjoyable longevity. Good health shouldn't mean giving up good food, or spending the rest of your long life obsessively counting calories. Intermittent fasting is a lifestyle that allows you to eat the way you like (up to a point!) while staying fit. In addition to that, scientific studies have shown that fasting can increase an animal's lifespan without retarding their growth, which is not the case for diets that focus on caloric restriction.

Chapter 2 - How Intermittent Fasting Works

The benefits of intermittent fasting are undeniably amazing, but before you are completely sold on adopting this lifestyle, you probably want to find out just why it's so effective for burning fat. What makes limiting the time that you eat any different from controlling your portions?

The fact is that intermittent fasting takes advantage of how your body naturally burns fat. The usual "six small meals a day" system aims to boost your metabolism under the principle that continually having a meal to burn off will keep your metabolic rates high as long as there is fuel for the fire, so to speak.

There is indeed some logic to this since burning a meal makes your body do quite a lot of work, butthe problem here is that your body will make use of the most readily available energy source – which would be the meal that you've just consumed. If you eat continuously, your body will never move on to burning fat. You'll actually end up storing more fat if you don't use up all the calories from your meals!

This is the opposite of what happens during fasting. After you've gone a certain number of hours without eating (the exact amount of time can vary from person to person), your body will have used up all the easily accessible calories from the last meal you ate, and it will have to start casting about for the next available energy source to burn to keep you going. And guess what? That next available energy source is the fat stored in your cells.

Yes, it really is that simple!

It's not just that, though. IF will also help you burn calories more efficiently even when you're not fasting by boosting the production of some hormones and normalizing your sensitivity to others.

For one thing, you are most sensitive to insulin when your energy stores have been depleted, such as after an intense workout or – you guessed it – a period of fasting. Increased sensitivity to insulin will help you burn the food you consume much more efficiently, leaving almost none of it to be stored as fat.

Human growth hormone (HGH) is also produced when your body is in a fasting state. This hormone is famously associated with fitness, and for good reason: it has the effect of helping build muscle mass while burning fat, which is, overall, the healthiest way to lose weight. Though shedding pounds is important, if you're doing it in such a way that you become weak and emaciated, you actually aren't doing yourself any favors in the long run.

It is, however, important to note that intermittent fasting is in no way equivalent to simply skipping a meal or taking things to the extreme and starving yourself. Skipping a meal and only waiting 3 or 4 hours before your next snack won't do anything except make you hungrier than ever (and thus more likely to binge).And starving yourself should

simply never be done: it is monumentally unhealthy to just stop eating and see how long you can go without taking a bite.

Intermittent Fasting works because you prepare yourself for the scheduled fasting period by consuming enough of the right kind of calories to keep you going beforehand, and you break your fast by having a good meal at the end of it.

Chapter 3 - Starting The Intermittent Fasting Lifestyle

So if it's not just a matter of skipping a meal or not eating for a day, what's the right way to start intermittent fasting?

To be perfectly honest, there is no universally prescribed protocol to begin your journey into the intermittent fasting lifestyle, as most experts on the subject will tell you. Different individuals will have varying needs when it comes to caloric intake and the amount of time it is possible to fast, and, as such, quite a number of IF schedules have been developed to suit the wide range of practitioners. However, since this book focuses on helping you get the best possible results from IF, we'll focus on daily intermittent fasting.

Daily intermittent fasting involves cycling the time that you eat (your feeding window) and the time that you abstain from food (the fasting period) within a 24-hour period. A lot of people start IF this way for a number of good reasons.

Firstly, the prospect of daily fasting is much less daunting than the idea of going a full 24 hours or more without food, especially for someone who's just coming off the "six small meals" paradigm that calls for constant eating. It's also a better option for somebody whose healthrequires the maintenance of certain blood sugar or metabolism levels. And it is simply easier to maintain than a weekly or alternate-day schedule since there is much less opportunity to let yourself fall off the wagon "just this once and it won't happen again".

Once you decide to start IF, it's essential to have a well thought-out plan of action before you start. Examine your schedule to see where you can place your feeding window and fasting period to maximize the effect without throwing you too far off your daily habits. For many people, the most comfortable time for the feeding window is from around noon to evening (1 PM to 8 PM, for example), or the time period that would normally encompass lunch and dinner.

This means that they get revved up by a calorie boost in the middle of the day and can comfortably go to bed on a full stomach. Yes, this also means that breakfast will be skipped, but, contrary to what we've all been taught since childhood, it is not absolutely necessary to a healthy lifestyle to start your day by loading up on calories.

Then you have to decide how long your feeding window and fasting period will be. It is generally agreed that the maximum length of a feeding window for effective IF is 8 hours, and that's probably where you should start. Adopting this on a daily schedule will mean that you can eat during 8 hours of a day and fast for the remaining 16 hours: a 16/8 scheme, or what is known as the Leangains model. If you are comfortable going for longer without eating, however, feel free to try 17/7, 18/6, 19/5, or even 23/1 schedules.

It might take you some time to find an IF schedule you are comfortable with, both in terms of the length of the feeding window and the time of day in which you place it. Feel free to experiment until you find the best fit for you, but once you've found it, you must make sure that you stick to it religiously. That is the only way that you'll see incredible results in just 7 days.

For the best results, you will have to integrate your workout into your intermittent fasting scheme so that you can take advantage of your new propensity to build muscle. Train 2 to 3 times a week, always scheduling your exercise sessions towards the end of your fasting period. That way, you'll burn your first big meal much more efficiently.

You will also have to carefully plan what you eat during the feeding window, and we'll talk about that in the next chapter.

Chapter 4 - What To Eat While On The Intermittent Fasting Diet

As has been said, just because intermittent fasting does not rely on counting calories does not mean that you can subsist solely on a diet of junk food during your feeding window. If you don't make at least some effort to eat healthy, IF will do nothing for you. But what should you eat to maximize the positive effects of fasting?

Focus on Protein and Veggies

During your feeding window, the main foods you should focus on are proteins and vegetables. This will ensure that you build up enough calories to see you through your fasting period while getting the nutrients you need.

One of the great things about intermittent fasting is that you're allowed a relatively large degree of freedom when it comes to your protein options. You can turn to meat, poultry, or fish, as long as they're prepared in a healthy manner. Consider grilled meats, baked fish, and turkey or chicken prepared in flavorful sauces redolent with exciting spices.

As for your vegetables, there are few things that will beat a salad made with garden-fresh greens. Try to get your veggies as fresh as possible so that you won't have to rely too much on salad dressings for the flavor. Healthy stews are also very much an option.

The Right Kind of Carbs

Unlike many other diet plans, intermittent fasting does not involve shunning all carbohydrates like the plague. In fact, it is strongly recommended that you eat a good portion of carbs on the days when you work out.

The trick, however, is sticking to the right kind of carbohydrates. Chips aren't a good idea, and neither is white bread. Go for rice (brown rice, for preference), quinoa, white bread, and oatmeal.

And if you're feeling the need to sink your teeth into something sweet for dessert, try fresh fruit instead of a slice of cake or bowl of ice cream. Go to your local farmer's market to see what's in season, or try more adventurous options like mango or dragon fruit if you want something more exciting.

Prepare Yourself for Big Portions

In intermittent fasting, it's not just what you eat – it's how much food you consume. You will have to prepare yourself to consume big portions during your feeding window. That way you'll avoid the common mistake of trying to fast on normal portions and ending up starving yourself because you didn't get enough calories.

This may come as a shock to you if you've just come off the "six small meals" way of thinking, but since you won't be eating as often, you have to make sure that you eat enough during the meals that you do consume. If you are daunted by the idea of having to eat so much food in one sitting, you can start by eating continuously when you're on your feeding window. But don't worry – when you stick to IF, you'll get used to sitting down for what looks like a giant meal.

Stay Hydrated While You Fast

Fasting does not mean that you should entirely refrain from letting anything pass your lips. During your fasting period, keep yourself hydrated by drinking plenty of water or fresh juice. Always have a bottle of something to drink on hand. Some people combine IF with herbal cleansing, which is a very sound idea.

Caffeinated drinks will also help, if you are still trying to get over the thought of cutting breakfast out of your life. Many IF practitioners swear by tea or coffee, especially since a cup of either-+r first thing in the morning will perk you up and help you feel less hungry. Go easy on the add-ons, though: you don't really need the whipped cream and chocolate syrup on your morning brew.

Occasionally Allow Yourself a Treat

Sticking to any diet can be difficult, and intermittent fasting, though easier than most, is no exception. Although you can eat a wide range of foods, it is undeniably frustrating not to be able to eat them whenever you want. For this reason, it's a good idea to allow yourself the occasional treat for good behavior.

You can, for instance, let yourself have a luxurious multi-scoop ice cream sundae for dessert after your last post-workout meal for the week. Or, following a week of strictly adhering to your intermittent fasting schedule, you could go out for dinner at your favorite restaurant and have those barbecue ribs you've been missing. Remember that while discipline is essential, it is equally important to keep yourself happy while you're on the road to fitness.

Chapter 5 - Tips And Tricks For Intermittent Fasting Success

Intermittent fasting is a simple and quick way to burn fat, but it comes with its own set of challenges. It can be hard to get used to, and if you go into it blindly, you might well give up and run for the fridge at the first onset of what you think are hunger pangs. To avoid that, and to help you stay on your IF schedule for 7 days, take note of these helpful tips and tricks.

Remember that Hunger is Mostly a State of Mind

The greatest challenge faced by people who try intermittent fasting is the mental block they encounter when they contemplate their prospective feeding habits. They look at the 16-hour fasting period and think that it's crazy to go completely without food for so long.

The first key for intermittent fasting success is thus to beat this unhelpful mindset. You've read this book, you've probably looked up numerous testimonials from confirmed fasters, so you know that you won't die of hunger on the IF diet. You also know that you don't actually need to eat continuously to go about your day. This hurdle can admittedly be the most difficult to overcome, but keep telling yourself that you can do it, and your body will follow.

Keep Yourself Occupied to Keep Your Mind Off Hunger

If you are having difficulty reminding yourself that hunger is mostly a state of mind, keep yourself occupied during your fasting period so that you do not constantly dwell on your hunger. This is why lots of practitioners favor the 1 PM to 8 PM feeding window: the resulting 16-hour is divided between sleep, and the busy first half of your working day. Find things to do to keep your mind off feeling hungry, and you'll be amazed at the sudden burst in your productivity.

If all else fails, however, you can resort to the old trick of keeping your mouth occupied while you're hungry. Chewing sugar-free gum is a classic standby, as is chewing ice cubes.

Don't Beat Yourself Up If You Go Off-Schedule

While strictly adhering to your schedule of feeding and fasting is a must for success, you mustn't beat yourself up if, for any reason, you go off schedule. Making yourself feel bad by dwelling on your transgression will not be helpful at all. If you lapse and do end up having that midnight snack, buck up and keep going. You will achieve much less if you give up on intermittent fasting at the first challenge you fail.

That being said, however, it's helpful to note that you don't have to adhere your IF scheme to the last minute or second. You don't have to stare longingly at your plate while you wait for the exact time of your fasting period to end if it's just a matter of 10 minutes or so.

Map Your Progress in a Diary

One of the things that will help you stay on track with intermittent fasting is mapping your progress in a diary or journal. For your initial 7-day trial of intermittent fasting, take note of your weight, and the percentage of your body fat. You will feel incredibly gratified when you see your results in a very real way as those numbers drop with every pound of fat that IF helps you burn.

You can also use the diary to plan out meals so that you don't have to hurriedly shop for the materials for a suitable meal every time your feeding window rolls around. And don't keep it clinical: write about how intermittent fasting makes you feel, how you deal with it, or just how much you are dying for a bag of chips if you think it'll help.

Seek Support from Others Who Do IF

You don't have to undertake intermittent fasting on your own. It's a wise idea to seek help from others who practice IF, and this is very easy to do. There are so many websites and forums that deal with this unique lifestyle, and the practitioners from all over the world tend to be very supportive of those who are new to the program. You can even give back to the IF community by sharing your own techniques, or turning your IF journal into a blog to show others that it's a great fitness option.

Conclusion

Thank you again for purchasing the book Intermittent Fasting!

I hope this book was able to help you understand, and more importantly, implement the principles of Intermittent Fasting to reach your fitness goals.

The next step is to get started using these strategies you have learned in this book and start becoming who you dream to be.

Also, if you know of anyone else that could benefit from the information presented here, please inform them about this book.

Finally, if you enjoyed this book, please take the time to share your thoughts and post a review on Amazon. It'd be greatly appreciated!

Thank you and good luck!

Preview Of:

<u>Fat Loss Secrets</u>

No Diets, No Supplements, Just Fat Loss Truth!

Introduction

I want to thank you and congratulate you for purchasing the book, "Fat Loss Secrets - No Diets, No Supplements, Just Fat Loss Truth!"

This book contains proven steps and strategies on how to lose fat and get the body you have always dreamed of!

Over the years, countless fad diets have come and gone. Along with the fad diets came the supplements. At first, some of the supplements seemed like they could be of benefit to you and healthy for you to consume, but as time has gone on so has the supplement industry. Supplements are now chemically engineered magic potion pills. Some of them do help you lose body fat, but at what expense to your health?

It doesn't have to be this complicated! If you are tired of riding the diet roller coaster and jumping on and off the hope train of the supplement industry, then you have come to the right place. This is where, armored with the truth, you can take control of your body and achieve your dreams for good. So read this book, apply the principles, and lose the fat.

Thanks again for purchasing this book, I hope you enjoy it!

Chris Smith

Chapter 1 - The Truth About Weight Loss

If you have ever thought about losing weight then you have
probably researched long and wide in search for the newest craze
to shed unwanted fat. If you have been taught by your weight loss
experience that skipping solid food and jogging a lot is the only
way to get the results that you want, you may be getting the entire
weight loss idea wrong.

The truth about weight loss is that it is not what it seems, and
people are getting the wrong kind of training when it comes to
what they should do to shed extra pounds. Here is the list of some
of the things that you thought are the sole reasons why people lose
weight.

- "Clean" and "detox" food.
- Excessive movement and exercise
- Staying away from junk food
- Lower sugar intake
- Lower amount of carbs in the diet
- Eating healthy food
- Refusing to eat dinner
- Doing cardio exercises
- Bodybuilding and gaining muscles
- Using a much smaller plate

These are just a few examples of an extensive list, but here's the
truth about these things. While they may assist in losing weight,
they are working on an entirely different concept, and so do you.
In fact, you can skip all these and still lose weight, which is
something that gym trainers and companies that sell healthy
packed juices, pills, and potions do not tell.

Losing weight does not need to be complicated or some sort of
rocket science, and even if you do not have the money to enroll in
a diet/nutrition program or gym training, the ideal weight is
achievable. All you need to do is pay attention to the calories that
you take in, it's really that simple! Crazy! Right? After all this
time we have been told that all food is not created equal, keep your
carbs and fats down and you will lose weight. I won't sit here and
tell you that eating vegetables and lean meats is not healthier for

you than eating sugar, carbs, and fats, but from a standpoint of losing weight, the most important thing you can do is take in less calories than you burn. That's it. If they exceed the requirement your body needs to function, shed them. In this sense, losing weight is actually very straightforward.

Thanks For Reviewing My Exciting Book Entitled:

"Fat Loss Secrets – No Diets, No Supplements, Just Fat Loss Truth!"

To purchase this book, simply go to the Amazon Kindle store and simply search:

"INTERMITTENT FASTING DIET"

Then just scroll down until you see my book. You will know it is mine because you will see my name "Chris Smith" underneath the title.

Alternatively, you can visit my author page on Amazon to see this book and other work I have done. Thanks so much, and please don't forget your free bonuses

DON'T LEAVE YET! - CHECK OUT YOUR FREE BONUSES BELOW!

Free Bonus Offer: Get Free Access To The www.LiveFitVIP.com VIP Newsletter!

Once you enter your email address you will immediately get free access to this awesome newsletter!

But wait, right now if you join now for free you will also get free access to the "The 7 Keys To Body Transformation" free EBook!

To claim both your FREE VIP NEWSLETTER MEMBERSHIP and your FREE BONUS EBook on THE 7 KEYS TO BODY TRANSFORMATION!

Just Go To:

www.liveFitVIP.com